Mahamadou Traoré
Bilaly Sissoko
Alkadri Diarra

Ureteral calculi at CHU Luxembourg Bamako

Mahamadou Traoré
Bilaly Sissoko
Alkadri Diarra

Ureteral calculi at CHU Luxembourg Bamako

Epidemiological and therapeutic aspects

ScienciaScripts

Imprint

Any brand names and product names mentioned in this book are subject to trademark, brand or patent protection and are trademarks or registered trademarks of their respective holders. The use of brand names, product names, common names, trade names, product descriptions etc. even without a particular marking in this work is in no way to be construed to mean that such names may be regarded as unrestricted in respect of trademark and brand protection legislation and could thus be used by anyone.

Cover image: www.ingimage.com

This book is a translation from the original published under ISBN 978-620-6-72118-5.

Publisher:
Sciencia Scripts
is a trademark of
Dodo Books Indian Ocean Ltd. and OmniScriptum S.R.L publishing group

120 High Road, East Finchley, London, N2 9ED, United Kingdom
Str. Armeneasca 28/1, office 1, Chisinau MD-2012, Republic of Moldova, Europe
Printed at: see last page
ISBN: 978-620-8-09628-1

DEDICATIONS AND THANKS

DEDICACES

To the Prophet Muhammad:

May ALLAH's blessing and peace be upon him. We show him our respect and gratitude.

To my country Mali,

Dear homeland, may peace and prosperity return to you. Deepest respect

To my father: Modibo TRAORE

This work is undoubtedly the fruit of the education you gave me and the immense sacrifices you made for my moral development; indeed, you were for us an example of courage, perseverance and honesty in the accomplishment of work well done. An exemplary father, you always fought to ensure that we lacked for nothing, so that we could study. You instilled in us the rules of good conduct, dignity, respect for human beings and wisdom. You are always there for us, sparing no effort or sacrifice so that we can benefit from a better education.

To my mother: Payi DOUCOURE

Sweet mother, unsurpassed woman, exemplary for your patience, courage, wisdom and devotion. You surrounded us with all your love, always protecting and comforting us. An irreproachable mother, you never for a moment ceased to care for our future with your many counsels and, above all, your blessings. Words cannot express my gratitude for all the sacrifices you endured to raise us. This modest work is the fruit of the sacrifices you made for my education and well-being. May ALLAH the Almighty grant you good health and a long life by our side. Amen!

To my mother: Adjarratou SIDIBE

As a hard-working, dignified woman, you spared no effort to ensure our success, and always comforted us in our most difficult moments.

I pray to ALLAH the All-Merciful to grant you health and prosperity.

To my uncle: the late Bourama TRAORE

(May God grant you his mercy, his paradise: amen!). You were truthful and kind, you always advised me how to behave with other people. I'll never forget you, sleep in peace!

To my uncle: Bakary TRAORE

You raised me to be rigorous and to succeed. Always concerned about our future, your moral and material support never failed me. You taught us to love and respect people, and to have the courage and stamina to face life. May this work bring you all the satisfaction you deserve.

ACKNOWLEDGEMENTS

A ALLAH :

Most Gracious, Most Merciful, Glory be to Allah, the Almighty, Creator of the heavens and the earth and all that lies between them, thank you for giving me life and watching over it, for giving me the health, the will, the courage and the strength to carry out this work. Help me through this training to save lives.

To the family of the late Salif Traoré :

And a special mention to the members of this family. You have made me your brother by keeping me in your family throughout my journey from high school to the end of this long cycle of medicine. May God give you peace and prosperity.

To all the Traoré family : Dioni ; Kénenkoun ; Bamako :

Thank you for everything you have done and continue to do. Words fail me to appreciate your gestures.

To the teaching staff of the DES in urology at the Faculty of Medicine and Odontostomatology in Bamako, and to all the teachers who have supported me in the teaching given.

To my brother Dr Moussa TRAORE:

Thank you for everything during this long journey. May Almighty God grant you a long and healthy life! Amen!

To my brothers and sisters:

Thank you for your unfailing support. Your sense of responsibility and love for one another reassures me. Please find here the expression of my affection and respect. May the Almighty ALLAH keep us united! We pray Amen!

To all my aunts, uncles and cousins

Please find here the expression of my deep gratitude. May God reward you all! Amen!

To my friends:

Thank you for your support. May ALLAH the Almighty strengthen our friendship! Amen!

To my fellow DES urology students, the eighth class of the FMOS numérus clausus; the Bouillagui FADIGA high school and the fundamental school Thank you for the moments spent together in mutual respect.

To all the staff of the urology departments of CHU Gabriel Touré, CHU du Point G, CHU de Kati and CHU Le Luxembourg

To all PhD students in the urology departments of CHU Gabriel Touré CHU du Point G, CHU de Kati and CHU Le Luxembourg

Thank you for your frank cooperation.

To all those, far and near, whose moral and financial support, however modest but how important to me, has made this modest work possible.

TRIBUTES TO JURY MEMBERS

To our master and jury president:

Professor Mamadou Lamine DIAKITÉ

> - **Urological Surgeon;**

> - **Full Professor of Urology at FMOS;**

> - **Head of the Urology Department at CHU du Point G ;**

> - **Director of Studies for the DES in Urology ;**

> - **President of the Malian Urology Association (AMUMALI).**

Dear master,

We're very grateful for the honor you've done us by agreeing to chair this jury, despite your busy schedule. Your human and intellectual qualities, your generosity and your availability have greatly impressed us. Your simplicity and your scientific qualities are examples to be followed. Please accept, dear Master, our deepest gratitude and sincere thanks.

To our master and judge:

Professor BERTHE Honoré Jean Gabriel

> - **Urological Surgeon;**

> - **Hospital practitioner at CHU du Point-G ;**

> - **Full Professor of Urology at FMOS;**

> - **Coordinator of the DES in Urology ;**

> - **General Secretary of the Association Malienne d'Urologie (AMU-MALI).**

Dear Master, we are very grateful for the honor you have bestowed on us by agreeing to judge our work. Your scientific rigor, your taste for work well done, your pedagogical and human qualities make you a definite hope for urology.

Please accept our sincere thanks.

To our master and judge:

Doctor COULIBALY Mamadou Tidiani

> **Urological Surgeon;**

> **Hospital practitioner at CHU Gabriel Touré ;**

> **Senior Lecturer in Urology at FMOS;**

> **Head of the Urology Department at CHU Gabriel TOURÉ ;**

> **Member of the Association Malienne d'Urologie (AMU-MALI).**

Dear master,

You have done us a great honor by agreeing to judge this work, despite your enormous workload. Your simplicity and availability make you a man of exceptional human qualities.

Please accept, dear master, the expression of our sincere admiration and deep gratitude.

To our master and thesis director:

Professor Alkadri DIARRA

> **Urological Surgeon;**

> **Hospital practitioner at the CHU Mère-Enfant Le Luxembourg ;**

> **Associate Professor of Urology at the FMOS ;**

> **Head of Urology at CHU Mère-Enfant Le Luxembourg ;**

> **President of the Conseil National de l'Ordre des Médecins du Mali.**

> **Member of the Association Malienne d'Urologie (AMU-MALI).**

Dear master,

We'll always remember you as a respectful, courageous and modest man. During our stay in the department, we were amazed by your way of working, you are undoubtedly a good framer, rigorous and very methodical. We are very grateful for the honour you have done us by agreeing to supervise this work, despite your busy schedule. Your scientific rigor, your availability and your ardent desire to pass on your extensive knowledge and technical skills to others make you a much-appreciated man of science.

TABLE OF CONTENTS

Table of contents

INTRODUCTION

I. INTRODUCTION

Ureteral iithiasis is defined as an aggregate of crystals in the ureteral excretory tract. They form and develop when excessive quantities of mineral salts, normally present in soluble form in the urine, crystallize.

It is a fairly widespread condition in the working population [1]. Caucasians and Eurasians have the highest stone prevalence rates, while Blacks, American Indians and Jews born in Israel have the lowest [2].

Today, urinary lithiasis is a widespread condition affecting between 4% and 18% of the population, depending on the country. On the increase in all industrialized countries, its frequency has almost doubled over the last half-century [2].

Elsewhere, the frequency of upper urinary tract lithiasis varies from country to country and region to region. Coffi U [3] in his 1973 study in Senegal, Adjanohoun [1] in 1989 in Benin and Diakité G.F [4] in 1985, Ongoïba I [5] in 1999 and Dembélé Z [7] in 2005, Coulibaly I [8] in Mali found respectively 39.1%; 38.1%; 43.4%; 43.8%; 44.45% and 15.65% of cases.

In our regions, specific conditions such as urinary bilharziasis or urogenital tuberculosis increase the incidence of ureteral lithiasis due to the ureteral lesions caused.

Urinary lithiasis is frequently recurrent and its etiopathogenesis is poorly understood, if not hypothetical [8].

Etiological investigation based on anamnestic, biological and radiological arguments, and biochemical analysis of the calculus, remains an essential element of the diagnosis, as lithiasis may be indicative of an underlying pathology. In most cases, the presence of a calculus will lead to obstruction.

The prognosis depends on whether the excretory tract and renal parenchyma are affected.

Its therapeutic challenges differ from those posed by kidney stones [3]. Like most urological conditions, urinary lithiasis is often discovered at the stage of complications [9].

This pathology is sometimes accompanied by extremely violent pain (renal colic) and microscopic or macroscopic haematuria [10]. The advent of endoscopic methods and extracorporeal lithotripsy has revolutionized the treatment of urinary lithiasis. However, in developing countries with limited technical resources, open surgery continues to be widely used in the management of urolithiasis [6]. Today, the urologist must decide on the best technique to use for each type of stone. However, the choice of which technique to use can be difficult, and depends on many factors:

• Calculus characteristics (number, size, location, composition and predictable hardness) ;

• characteristics of the excretory tract (associated anatomical anomaly, dilatation, ureteral stenosis);

• patient characteristics (age, weight, morphotype, general condition, etc.) ;

• technical platform and operator habits (presence of a fixed or mobile lithotripter, availability and quality of endo-urological equipment, etc.)

For the treatment of pelvic ureter stones, ureteroscopy (URS) is essential and, together with extracorporeal lithotripsy (ECL), represents the two first-line treatments.

Fourier Transform Infrared Spectroscopy (FTIR) is the method of choice due to its versatility, rapid determination of stone composition and structure, and low cost. This analysis provides an orientation towards the pathology responsible for stone formation, and thus indicates to the clinician the first therapeutic measure to be considered in lithiasis sufferers [7].

OBJECTIVES

II.   OBJECTIVES

2.1. GENERAL OBJECTIVE

Study the epidemiological and therapeutic aspects of ureteral iithiasis at the University Hospital of Luxembourg

2.2. SPECIFIC OBJECTIVES

1. Determine the frequency of ureteral lithiasis

2. Describe clinical and evolutionary aspects

3. Describe the therapeutic aspects of ureteral lithiasis

METHODOLOGY

III. METHODOLOGY

1. Type and location of study :

This was a retrospective descriptive study of a series of patients presenting with ureteral lithiasis in the urology department of C.H.U le Luxembourg.

2. Study period :

Our study was spread over a 6-year period, from January 2017 to December 2022.

3. Inclusion criteria:

All patients treated for ureteral lithiasis during the study period were included in this study.

4. Non-inclusion criteria:

Patients with urinary lithiasis outside the period and non-lithiasis patients were not included.

5. Data entry and processing :

Data were collected using Cinzan software.

Data entry and analysis on SPSS software

Tables and figures were created using Word and Excel 2010.

6. Parameters studied :

- Anamnestic data: patient's identity, medical and surgical history.

- Clinical data: symptomatology.

- Paraclinical data: radiological and biological workup.

- Lithiasis characteristics: size, number, location, density, etc.

- Management and therapeutic results.

RESULTS

IV. RESULTS

1. FREQUENCY :

During the study period, 985 surgical procedures were performed out of 3020 consultations, i.e. 32.61%. 75 patients consulted for ureteral calculi, i.e. 2.48% of the department's activities, 67 patients were treated surgically, i.e. 6.80% of the department's surgical activities. Of the 75 patients treated for ureteral calculi: 8 patients underwent expulsive medical treatment, 23 patients underwent open ureterolithotomy surgery and 44 patients underwent ureteroscopy.

2. SOCIO-DEMOGRAPHIC ASPECTS :

2-   1. Age :

Table I: Patient distribution by age group

Age range	Workforce	Percentage	cumulative
inf 12 years	2	2,7	2,7
12 - 24 years	9	12,0	14,7
25 - 37 years	26	34,7	49,3
38 - 50 years	**27**	**36,0**	**85,3**
Sup 50 years	11	14,7	100

The 38-50 age group was the most represented.

The mean age of patients was **37.32** years, with extremes ranging from **10 to 75** years and a standard deviation of **12.18** years.

2-2. Gender:

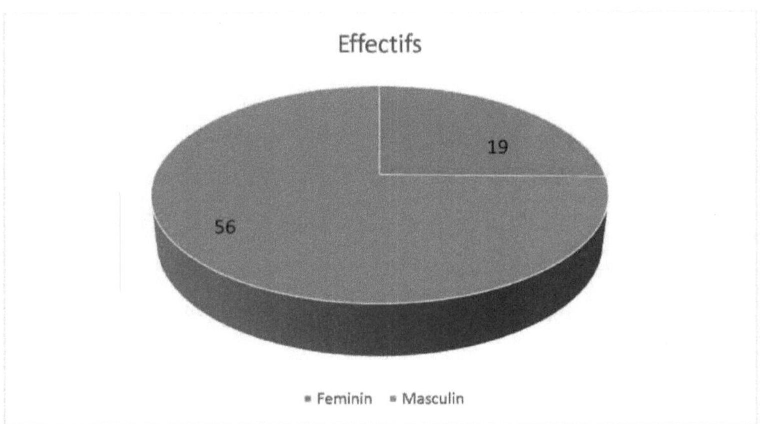

Figure 1: Distribution of patients by gender.

The male gender was the most represented, with 56 cases.

CLINICAL ASPECTS

3-   1. Reason for consultation :

Table II: Breakdown by reason for consultation

Reason for consultation	Workforce	Percentage	% Cumulative
Lumbago	50	66,67%	65,3
Hematuria	1	1,33%	66,7
pollakiuria	1	1,33%	68,0
Hypogastric pain	4	5,33%	73,3
RR for calculation	18	24,00%	97,3
RR for left hydronephrosis	1	1,33%	98,7
Total	**75**	**100,00%**	**100%**

Low back pain was the main reason for consultation with **50 patients**, i.e. **66.67%**.

4. ADDITIONAL EXAMINATIONS :

4-   1. BIOLOGY :

a. Creatinine levels :

Table III: Distribution of patients by renal function

Creatinine	Workforce	Percentage	cumulative
Less than 60µmol/l	13	17,33	17,33
60 to 120µmol/l	35	46,67	64
Sup to 120µmol/l	27	36,00	100
Total	**75**	**100**	

Renal function was elevated in 27 patients, or 36%.

b. Cytobacteriological examination of urine

Table IV: Distribution of patients according to germs

ECBU	Workforce	Percentage	% accumulates
Negative	60	80%	80
E. Coli	**7**	**9,33%**	**89, 33**
K. pneumo	5	6,67%	96
Pseudomonas	3	4%	100
Total	**75**	**100%**	

Urine cytobacteriological examination (UCE) was culture positive in 15 patients (20%). The most frequently found germ was Escherichia coli (7/15).

4-2. Imaging :

Imaging performed

Table V: Distribution of patients according to imaging diagnostic method

Imaging	Workforce	percentage
Ultrasound	1	1,3
Uroscanner	74	98,7
Total	75	100,0

CT scanning was the main imaging test performed.

Location of calculations :

Table VI: Distribution of patients according to uroscanner stone location

Calculation_Location	Workforce	Percentage	%cumulated
Right lumbar ureter	26	34,7	34,7
Right Iliac Ureter	4	5,3	40,0
Right pelvic ureter	13	17,3	57,3
Left pelvic ureter	7	9,3	66,7
Left Iliac Ureter	2	2,7	69,3
Uretere ilaque Left	2	2,7	72,0
Left Lumbar Uretere	12	16,0	88,0
left ureteral meatus	3	4,0	92,0
Right pyloric region	1	1,3	93,3
Right ureterovesical junction	5	6,7	100,0
Total	**75**	**100,0**	

Lithiasis was localized in the lumbar region (38cas), with a right-sided predominance.

Number of calculations :

Table VII: Distribution of patients by number of calculations

Calculation_Number	Workforce	Percentage	cumulative
1	69	92,0	92
2	6	8,0	100
Total	**75**	**100,0**	

The number of stones in the same patient was 1(69 patients)

Calculation size :

Table VIII: Distribution of patients by stone size

Size (mm)	Workforce	Percentage
Below 7	17	22,7
7 - 10	16	21,3
11 - 20	33	44,0
Sup à 20	9	12,0
Total	**75**	**100,0**

Lithiasis density :

Table IX: Distribution of patients according to lithiasis density

Density (UH)	Workforce	Percentage	cumulative
Under 500	22	29,3	29,3
500 - 1000	28	37,3	66,6
Above 1000	25	33,3	100
Total	**75**	**100,0**	

4. THERAPEUTIC ASPECTS

4-1. Processing methods:

Table X: Breakdown of patients by treatment mode

Treatment	Workforce	Percentage	cumulative
Expulsive medical treatment	8	10,7	10,7
Ureterolithotomy	24	32,0	42,7
Ureteroscopy	**41**	**54,7**	**97,4**
Meat resection	2	2,6	100
Total	**75**	**100,0**	

Ureteroscopy was performed in **54.7%** of patients

4-2. Drainage methods :

Table XI: Distribution of patients according to drainage mode :

JJ fitting	Workforce	Percentage
Yes	63	84,0
No	12	16,0
Total	**75**	**100**

JJ catheterization was performed in 84% of patients.

4-3. JJ removal time :

Table XII: Distribution of patients by JJ removal time :

JJ removal	Workforce	Percentage
1 month	**54**	**85,7**
2 months	7	11,1
3 months	2	3,2
Total	**63**	**100**

JJ removal was performed at 1 month postoperatively in 85.7% of cases.

6. EVOLUTIONARY ASPECT

6-1. Repeat:

Table XIII: Distribution of patients according to the occurrence of recurrence

Recurrence	Workforce	Percentage
Yes	3	4
No	72	96
Total	**75**	**100**

The recurrence rate was 4%.

Table XIV: Results by treatment mode

Results/ Treatment.	Satisfied		Not satisfied		Total	
	Workforce	%	Workforce	%	Workforce	%
Expulsive medical treatment	4	50	4	50	8	10,7
Ureterolithotomy	23	96	1	4	24	32,0
Ureteroscopy	**40**	**98**	**1**	**2**	**41**	**54,7**
Meat resection	2	100	0	0	2	2,6
Total	69	92	6	8	75	100,0

Patient satisfaction with ureteroscopy was **98%**.

COMMENTS AND DISCUSSION

V. COMMENTS AND DISCUSSION

1. EPIDEMIOLOGICAL ASPECTS

1.1 Frequency :

During the study period, **75** patients consulted for ureteral calculi, representing 2.48% of the department's activity.

Elsewhere, the frequency of upper urinary tract lithiasis varies from country to country and region to region. Coffi U [3] in his 1973 study in Senegal, Adjanohoun [1] in 1989 in Benin and Diakité G.F [4] in 1985, Ongoïba I [5] in 1999 and Dembélé Z [7] in 2005, Coulibaly I [8] in Mali found respectively 39.1%; 38.1%; 43.4%; 43.8%; 44.45% and 15.65% of cases.

1.2 Age :

The average age of patients was **37.32** years, with extremes of 10 and 75 years. The 38-50 age group was the most affected, at 36%.

Studies similar to ours by Yatarra I. [6] , Keita O. [11], Sangaré Y. [12] and Dembélé Z. [7] reported the same results.

These results show that the age group most frequently affected by urinary lithiasis corresponds to the period of genital and professional activity.

1.3 Gender :

The male sex was the most represented, with 74.66% of cases. This result is close to that of Coulibaly I. [8], Traoré B [14], Sohel H. A [15], Zoung K J and Sow M [9], Daffé S I [19], Diakité G F [4], Sangaré Y [12], who recorded 72%; 88.43%; 88% 86.44%; 81.09%; 79.25%; 73.8% respectively. This male predominance can be explained by the fact that men are more exposed to bilharzian infestation than women, but also by organic factors that can favor lithogenesis in men (urethral stricture, prostatic hypertrophy, sclerosis of the bladder neck).

2. CLINICAL ASPECTS

2.1 Reason for consultation :

We noted that back pain was the main symptom in over 66.67% of our patients.

Traoré Y.N. [16] and Coulibaly M. [17] found 83% and 79.24% respectively of low back pain.

2.2 Creatinine levels:

The simplest and most reliable test, whose elevation is indicative of impaired renal function, which can progress to renal failure.

In our study, we found that 36% of patients had renal impairment (moderate or severe). This result is superior to those of Yattara I. [6]; Sangaré Y. [12] and Ouédraogo I. [20], who had 16.1%; 6.22% and 8.96% respectively. This could be explained by the more frequent unilateral nature of ureteral lithiasis.

2.3 Urine cytobacteriological examination (ECBU):

It was performed on all patients. The culture was sterile in 80% of cases. Escherichia coli was isolated in **9.33%** of cases. This result differs from those of Daffé S I. [19], Ongoïba I. [5], Sangaré Y. [12], Dembélé Z. [7]

and Sohel H B. [15], who respectively found 79.05%; 52.2%; 42.9%; 35.2% and 28.12% cases of urinary tract infection.

This result can be explained by the fact that most patients self-medicate with antibiotics.

2.4 Imaging :

All our patients underwent a radiological examination. Radiological examinations (ultrasound and CT scan) play an important role in the management of urinary lithiasis.

In our study, there was a predominance of the right side (57.3% on the right versus 42.7% on the left). This result differs from that of Pérou A. [20], who found a frequency of 37% on the right and 35.6% on the left.

The number of stones in the same patient in our study varied from 1 to 2 stones.

3. THERAPEUTIC ASPECTS

Ureteral lithiasis is treated by open surgery, extracorporeal lithotripsy and ureteroscopy. Minimally invasive techniques offer interesting results, with very simple post-operative follow-up.

In our series, ureteroscopy was the most commonly used curative treatment in 54.7% of cases.

This result differs from that of Coulibaly I. [8] and Yattara I. [6], who performed more open surgery for lithiasis.

4. EVOLUTIONARY ASPECT

Recurrence was found in 4% of patients in our study In the absence of preventive measures, recurrence of a urinary calculus is almost inevitable. It is estimated that the risk of recurrence is 30-40% at five years, and 50-70% at ten years. Recurrence is more likely if the disease began in a young person (before the age of 30 or 40). The risk factors are essentially linked to our dietary habits, which today are too rich in proteins, salt, sugar, fats and soft drinks, and too low in fruit, vegetables and dairy products [20].

CONCLUSION AND RECOMMENDATIONS

VII. CONCLUSION AND RECOMMENDATIONS

1. Conclusion:

Ureteral lithiasis is quite common in hospital practice in the urology department of CHU Le Luxembourg.

It occurs in the working population. It can be seen at any age, and more frequently in males.

Ureteral calculi, like all other urinary tract lithiasis, are responsible for temporary professional incapacity. As a result, it is a cause of absenteeism, and therefore of lost working days.

The most common symptoms are low back pain or attacks of renal colic.

The radiological work-up, based essentially on Uroscanner, revealed calculi in all cases.

Management is multidisciplinary. Technological advances, in particular the miniaturization of endoscopes and the performance of fragmentation techniques, have facilitated management, especially of small stones, which tend to recur.

2. RECOMMENDATIONS :

❖ To the public:

- Seek prompt medical attention for any pain or difficulty urinating.

❖ To healthcare personnel:

- Prompt referral to specialized services.

- Maintain close collaboration with other departments to facilitate interdepartmental transfers.

❖ To the political and health authorities:

- Training urologists.

- The opening of a local urinary stone analysis center.

- Launch NLPC and laser ureteroscopy in urology departments.

BIBLIOGRAPHICAL REFERENCES

VII. BIBLIOGRAPHICAL REFERENCES

1. Adjanohoun F. J

Urinary lithiasis in the surgical services of the CNHU of Cotonou: 109 cases observed in 18 years. Thesis, Cotonou, 1989, N°427.

2. Hannache B.

Urinary lithiasis: Epidemiology, role of trace elements and medicinal plants. Human medicine and pathology. Université Paris Sud - Paris XI, 2014. French. NNT: 2014PA114804. Doctoral thesis. N°01261

3. URBAN COFFI M. A.

Contribution à l'étude de la lithiase urinaire chez l'africain au Sénégal à propos de 123 observations. Méd. thesis, Dakar, 1981, No. 15.

4. DIAKITE G.F.

Urinary **lithiasis** in hospitals in Bamako about 53 cases. Thesis.

Bamako, 1985, No. 21.

5. Ongoïba I.

Lithiasis of the urinary tract in the urology department of the HNPG. Thèse Med 1999. N°92

6. Yattara I.

Adult urinary lithiasis in the urology department of CHU Point G: Epidemiological, clinical, para-clinical and therapeutic aspects. Mémoire Med 2021.

7. Dembélé Z.

Epidemiology and treatment of urinary lithiasis in the urology department of Point G National Hospital. Thèse Med 2005. N°05M55

8. Coulibaly I.

Ureteral lithiasis: Clinical aspects diagnostic and therapeutic approach in the urology department of CHU Gabriel TOURE. Thesis Med 2014. N°14M96

9. Zoung-Kanyi J., Sow M.

Urinary lithiasis in Cameroon etiopathogenic, clinical and therapeutic considerations. A propos de 118 cas. Médecine d'Afrique Noire: 1990, 37 (4): 176182

10. Odzebe ASW, Bouya PA, Berthe HJG, Omatassa FR.

Open surgery for urinary lithiasis at Brazzaville University Hospital: analysis of 68 cases. Mali médical 2010; XXV (2): 32-35

11. Keïta O.

Study of infected urinary lithiasis in the urology department of the Point G university hospital. Thesis Med 2006.

12. Sangaré Y.

Urinary lithiasis in Point hospital urology departments

G and Gabriel Touré. Mémoire Med 2015.

13. Cissé Soriba

"Semi-rigid ureteroscopy at CHU Luxembourg". PhD Thesis, USTTB, 2020.

14. Traoré B

Contribution à l'étude épidémiologique des lithiases urinaires dans les Hôpitaux de Bamako et de Kati à propos de 95 cas. Thesis, Bamako, 1984, N°35.

15. Sohel H A

Urinary lithiasis in children: 60 cases. Med. thesis, Dakar, 1981, N°21.

16. Traore Y.N.

Study of urinary tract lithiasis in the urology department of CHU du G-spot: about 100 cases. Thesis Med 2012. N°13M10

17. Coulibaly M

Study of lithiasis of the upper urinary tract in the urology department of the CHU du Point G: A propos de 53 cases. Thèse Med 2007. N°07M122

18. Ouédraogo I., Madina A.N., Bandre E., Ouédraogo S., Tapsoba W.T., Wandraogo A.

Urinary calculi in children in Burkina Faso: about 67 cases. Pan African Medical Journal. 2015 ; 20 :352

[doi: 10.11604/pamj.2015.20.352.4407]

19. Daffé S I

Urinary lithiasis in the Republic of Mali: 132 cases. Thesis, Bamako, 1989, N°38.

20. PEROU A.

Contribution of imaging in the diagnosis of urinary lithiasis.

Thesis Med. 2003. N°03M86

21. https:/ampsante.lefigaro.fr/actualite/2011/06/05/10915-comment-peut-on- éviter-recidive-calculsurinaires.

APPENDICES

TITLE: Ureteral lithiasis in the urology department of CHU Le Luxembourg: epidemiological and therapeutic aspects.

City of defense: Bamako

Country of origin: Mali

Sector of interest: Urology

Depository: Library of the Faculty of Medicine and Odontostomatology of Mali.

Summary:

Title: Les lithiases urétérales dans le service d'urologie du CHU Le Luxembourg: Aspects épidémiologiques, et thérapeutiques.

Objective: To study the epidemiological and therapeutic aspects of ureteral lithiasis at the University Hospital of Luxembourg.

Methodology: This was a retrospective descriptive study of a series of patients with ureteral lithiasis over a 6-year period, from January 2017 to December 2022 in the urology department of C.H.U le Luxembourg.

Results :

➢ The frequency of ureteral lithiasis is 2.48%.

➢ The 38-50 age group was the most affected, with extremes of 10 and 75.

➢ The sex ratio was 2.95 in favor of men.

➢ Pain was the main symptom, followed by urinary disorders and haematuria.

➢ Ureteral iithiases also play an important role in impaired renal function and urinary tract infections.

➢ Radiological examinations play an important role in the management of urinary lithiasis.

➢ Ureteroscopy was used as curative treatment in 54.7% of cases.

Conclusion:

Ureteral lithiasis is quite common in hospital practice in the urology department of CHU Le Luxembourg.

In our study, it was more common in the working population, with a male predominance.

Endoscopic surgery has played an important role.

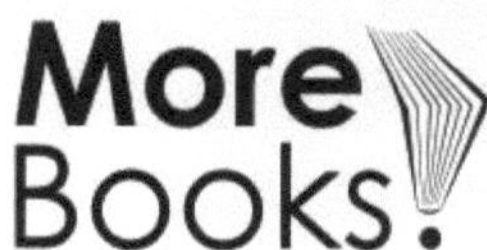

More
Books!

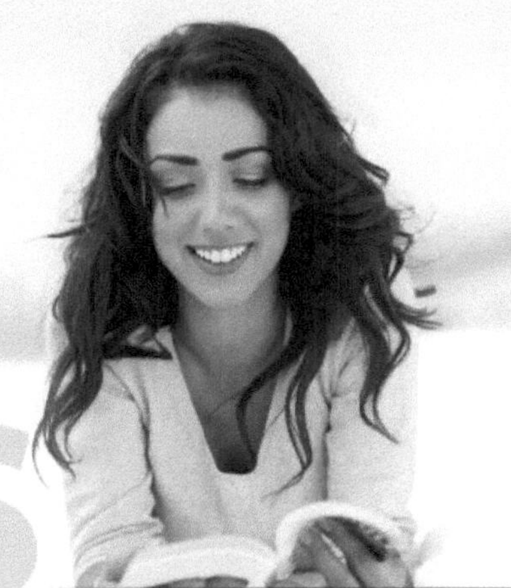

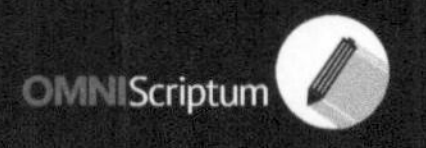

info@omniscriptum.com
www.omniscriptum.com
OMNIScriptum

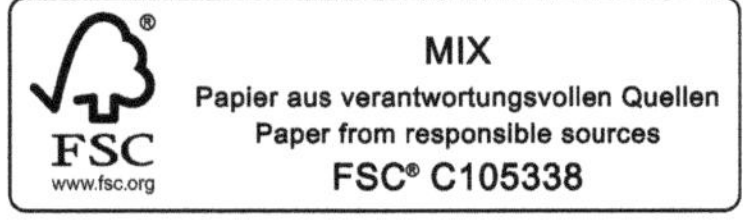

Printed by Books on Demand GmbH, Norderstedt / Germany